The Teen Mom Survival Guide

A step by step guide for teen Mum

Cordelia R. Cole

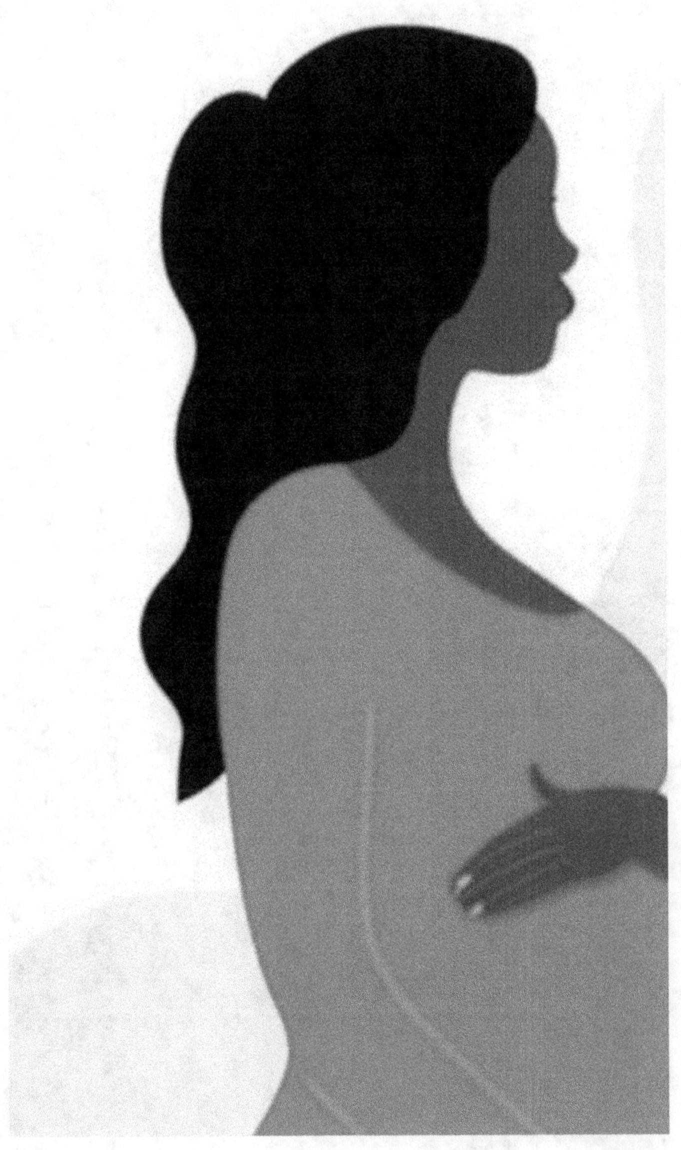

Table Of Content

- **Encouragement and Support for Your Future**

Introduction

The Teen Mom's Survival Guide is a comprehensive resource for teen moms dealing with the challenges of motherhood. We offer young mothers practical advice and support with challenges ranging from financial difficulties to emotional and psychological stress.

This guide covers a wide range of topics including prenatal care, childbirth, breastfeeding, postpartum recovery, and parenting. It also covers topics such as education, career planning, and financial management, which are essential for teen mothers to build a stable and secure future for themselves and their children.

In addition to practical advice, the Survival Guide for Teen Moms offers emotional support for young moms who feel overwhelmed or isolated. Includes tips on building a support network, managing stress and anxiety, and overcoming the challenges of being a single parent.

Overall, the Teen Mom's Survival Guide is a valuable resource for teen moms looking for advice and support as they navigate the complex and rewarding journey of motherhood.

Chapter One

My path as a teenage mother

As the author of this book, I am a proud teen mom who has been through a lot along the way. When I found out I was pregnant at a young age, I was scared and unsure of what the future held for me. Like many teen moms, I faced a variety of challenges, from the emotional turmoil of an unplanned pregnancy to the practical difficulties of balancing motherhood with school and other commitments.

But despite the challenges, I never lost sight of my dreams and goals. With the support of my loved ones and my own inner strength, I was able to overcome the obstacles in my path and build a better life for myself and my son.

My journey as a teen mom has taught me many valuable lessons about resilience, perseverance, and the power of a positive mindset. I have learned that despite adversity there is always hope for a better future. By setting realistic goals, seeking sources of support, and focusing on what matters most, I've been able to build a life I'm proud of.

In this book, I want to share my own experiences as a teen mother while providing practical advice, ideas, and inspiration for others facing similar challenges. Whether you're struggling with an unexpected pregnancy, struggling to balance motherhood and school, or just looking for guidance and support on your journey through teen motherhood, this book is for you.

Together we can harness the power of resilience and perseverance and

create a better, more fulfilling future for
ourselves and our children.

What is teenage pregnancy?

A teenage pregnancy is defined as a pregnancy in a woman under the age of 19. It is a major public health problem affecting individuals, families and communities around the world. Teenage pregnancy rates vary widely between countries, but are more common in low- and middle-income countries than in high-income countries.

There are several factors that can contribute to teenage pregnancy, including lack of access to sex education, limited knowledge of birth control methods, poverty, peer pressure, and low self-esteem. In some cases, teenage pregnancy can also be the result of sexual abuse or sexual exploitation.

Teenage pregnancy can have significant physical, emotional and social consequences for both mother and child. Teenage mothers are more likely to experience complications during pregnancy and childbirth, such as preterm birth and low birth weight. They are also more likely to drop out of school, have limited career opportunities and face financial difficulties.

Children of teenage mothers can also face major challenges such as:poor health, developmental delays and limited access to resources and support. They are also more likely to be poor and less educated than children of older mothers.

Despite the challenges associated with teenage pregnancy, resources and support are available to help young mothers navigate the experience. Access to comprehensive sex education, birth control, and prenatal care can help reduce teen pregnancy rates and improve maternal and child outcomes. Support from family, friends, and caregivers can also help young mothers succeed as parents and achieve their goals.

Teen Pregnancy Causes

Teenage pregnancy can result from a variety of factors, including social, economic, and cultural influences. Here are some common causes of teen pregnancy:

1. Lack of access to sex education: Many teens do not have access to comprehensive sex education on topics such as birth control, pregnancy, and sexually transmitted diseases. Without this knowledge, teens may not

know how to prevent pregnancy or understand the consequences of sexual activity.

2. Limited knowledge of birth control methods: Even if teens have access to birth control, they may not know how to use it effectively. They may also have misconceptions about birth control, believing it to be ineffective or harmful.

3. Peer Pressure: Teens may feel pressured by their peers to

engage in sexual activity, especially if they believe it is normative behaviour among their friends.

4. Low self-esteem: Teens with low self-esteem may engage in sexual activity to gain confidence or seek validation from others.

5. Poverty: Teens from low-income households may be at greater risk of pregnancy due to limited access to resources

such as birth control and sex education.

6. Lack of parental involvement: Adolescents who lack parental involvement and supervision are more likely to engage in sexual activity and are less likely to use birth control.

7. Sexual Abuse or Exploitation: In some cases, a teenage pregnancy can be the result of sexual abuse or exploitation by a partner, family member, or stranger.

Reducing the incidence of teenage pregnancy requires a multifaceted approach that addresses these root causes. This can include improving access to comprehensive sex education and contraception, tackling poverty and inequality, promoting healthy relationships and self-esteem, and tackling sexual abuse and exploitation.

The challenges of teenage pregnancy

Teenage pregnancy can be a challenging experience for both mother and child. Here are some common challenges that teenage moms can face:

1. Physical Health Complications: Teenage mothers are at higher risk of physical health complications during pregnancy and childbirth, such as:

premature birth, low birth weight and pregnancy-related high blood pressure.

2. Emotional Health Challenges: Teenage pregnancies can be emotionally draining, and teenage mothers are at higher risk of developing postpartum depression and anxiety. They may also experience feelings of isolation and loneliness as their peers may not

understand the challenges of raising children at a young age.

3. Financial Issues: Teenage mothers can face financial issues, including the cost of medical care, childcare, and the child's basic needs. They may also have limited earning potential due to limited education and work experience.

4. Social Stigma and Discrimination: Teenage mothers can face social stigma and discrimination, which can lead to feelings of shame and isolation. They may also face judgement and criticism from peers, family members, and community members.

5. Limited educational opportunities: Teenage mothers may be at greater risk of dropping out of school

or delaying their education due to the demands of parenthood. This can limit their career opportunities and long-term earning potential.

6. Limited Support: Teenage mothers may not have access to adequate support from family members, friends, or caregivers. This can make it difficult to deal with the challenges of parenthood at a young age.

Despite these challenges, resources and support are available to help teenage mothers overcome these obstacles. Prenatal care, counselling, and parenting classes can help teenage mothers prepare for parenthood and cope with the emotional challenges of pregnancy and parenthood. Financial aids such as government programs and community organisations can also cover the cost of childcare and the child's basic needs. Finally, social support from family members, friends, and caregivers can help teenage mothers feel supported and less isolated.

Chapter 2

Decision to become a teenage mama

Becoming a parent can be challenging at any age, but becoming a parent as a teen comes with unique challenges. Deciding to become a teen mama is a life- changing decision that requires a lot of study, medication, and support. In this chapter, we'll look at some of the factors that go into deciding to become a teen mama and the ways you can prepare for that responsibility.

Understanding Parenthood liabilities

Becoming a parent means accepting the responsibility for life to watch for and support another mortal being. As a teen parent, you're responsible for your child's physical, emotional, and financial needs. This responsibility requires time, tolerance and sacrifices. Before you decide to become a teen parent, it's important to understand the full compass of that responsibility and what it means for your life.

**Considering your options
Adoption, Abortion or
Parenting**

Faced with an unanticipated gestation, you have three main options Abortion, Adoption or parenting. Each option has its unique benefits and challenges, and it's important to precisely estimate each option before making a decision.

1. Abortion / Revocation is a medical procedure that ends a gestation. It's a veritably particular decision that requires careful consideration of your beliefs, values, and circumstances.However, it's important to speak with a health care provider pertaining to your options and make an informed decision, If

you're considering an
revocation.

2. Adoption/Relinquishment
is a legal process in which
you freely give up your
maternal rights to your
child. It's a decision that
requires a lot of study and
consideration, but it can
give your child a stable
and lovinghome.However,
it's important to work with

a estimable relinquishment/adoption agency and seek advice so that you can make the stylish decision for you and your child, If you're considering relinquishment.

3. Parenthood is an important responsibility that requires time, tolerance, and

sacrifice.However, it's important to prepare yourself for the challenges that come with that responsibility, If you decide to become a teen mama .

Erecting A Strong Support System

Seeking antenatal care, and planning for your child's future are important ways in preparing for parenting. Becoming a teen mama can be segregating, but erecting a strong support system can make all the difference. A support system can include your family,health care providers, and other teen mothers who understand what you're going through. It's important to communicate your needs and ask for help when you must. Remember that it takes a city to raise a child and erecting a strong support system is critical to your success as a teen mama .

Dealing With The Emotional Impact Of A Teen Gestation

Dealing with the emotional impact of a teen gestation requires admitting and addressing the passions and enterprises that arise during this time. Here are some strategies that can help

- Seek support: Talk to someone you trust, similar as a parent, friend, or counsellor, about your passions and enterprises. They can offer emotional support and guidance.

- Get informed: Learn all you can about pregnancy, and parenthood. This can help you be more set and more confident in conforming to your situation.

- Take care of your physical health: eat well, rest and exercise regularly. This can help you feel more physically and emotionally.

- Consider your options about your pregnancy options, similar to parenting, Adoption, or Abortion.

- Talk to a health care provider or counsellor to help you make an informed decision.

- Plan for the future Set objectives and make a plan for your future, including educational, career, and family goals. This can help you to break through

Chapter 3

Navigate Your Gestation

Navigating gestation as a teenage mama can be inviting. In this chapter, we examine the methods you can take to put up with your body, prepare for labour and delivery, and address common gestation symptoms and enterprises.

Handling Your Body

Antenatal Care and Nutrition

Antenatal care is essential for both your health and the soundness of your baby. It's important that you seek antenatal care as soon as possible after you find out you're pregnant. Antenatal care includes regular check-up with a health care provider, tests and examinations to check the fitness of you and your baby, and education about gestation and parturition. When looking for antenatal care, it's vital to find a provider that you feel comfortable with and has experience working with teenage mothers.

Your healthcare provider can cover your gestation and address your enterprises. They may also offer you fresh support coffers, similar as Counselling services or educational courses. In addition to antenatal care, it's important to take care of your body with the right diet. Eating a balanced diet high in fruits, vegetables, whole grains, and spare protein can help keep your growing baby healthy. It's also important to avoid certain foods and substances that can harm your baby, similar to alcohol, tobacco, and medicines. Good nutrition is essential during gestation. In addition to a balanced diet, you may need to take an antenatal.

Vitamins to insure you are getting enough nutrients like folic acid. Your health insurance company will advise you on good nutrition and salutary supplements.

Dealing with common gestation complaints and Concern

Dealing with the symptoms and Concern of gestation can be challenging for any mama - to- be. Gestation can bring with it a variety of symptoms and concerns, including morning sickness, fatigue, back pain and further, but as a teenage mama, you may have other concerns related to your age and experience. hitherto are some tips for dealing with gestation symptoms and concern as a teenage mama.

- Talk to a Healthcare Provider: It's important to have an antenatal care from a health care provider during gestation. They can help you cover your health and that of your baby, answer your questions, and give support and guidance.
- Eat a healthy diet: A balanced and nutritional

diet is important for both your health and that of your baby. Make sure you include an abundance of fruits, vegetables, spare proteins, and whole grains in your diet.

- Get abundance of rest: Is important during gestation, so make sure you get enough sleep and take breaks when you need them.

- Stay active: Regular exercise during gestation can enhance your health and reduce some of the discomforts of gestation. Consult your Crocker before beginning any new exercise program.

- Address parenthood Concern If you have Concern about being a good parent, it can help to seek out coffers and support. This could include attending parenthood classes, connecting with other teenage mothers, or working with a therapist. Remember that gestation symptoms and Concern are normal and it's okay to ask for help and support when you need it. With the right care and support, you can have a healthy gestation and a successful transition into parenthood

Preparing for childbearing and delivery

Preparing for labour and delivery is an important part of your gestation. It's important to take parturition education classes, which can give you information about the different stages of labor, pain handling tactics, and more. You'll also need to bring about a birth plan detailing your labour and delivery preferences. Nonetheless, it's important to visit the clinic and meet your Doctor and clinic staff to ensure you're set for the big day, if you're planning to give birth in a hospital.

However, similar to For illustration, if you're having a home birth or a birth centre, if you have indispensable birth options.

As a teenage mom, preparing for childbirth and having children can be overwhelming, but it's important to take the necessary steps to ensure a healthy pregnancy and birth. however here are some advice to keep in mind:

- Prenatal care: Prenatal care is essential to a healthy pregnancy and birth. Schedule regular checkups with your physician to monitor your health and your baby's growth.

- Eat a healthy diet: Eating a healthy, balanced diet is important for both you and your baby. Make sure you're getting enough nutrients, including folic acid, iron, and calcium.

- Stay Active: Staying active during pregnancy can help you stay healthy and reduce your risk of complications. Talk to your medic about what types of exercises are safe for you.

- Take antenatal classes: antenatal classes can help you prepare for labour and delivery and give you the tools you need to manage pain and stress during the process.

- Prepare for postpartum recovery: Postpartum, your body needs time to recover. Make sure you have a postpartum care plan in place, including support from family and friends and access to any necessary medical services.

- Find Emotional Support: Becoming a mother to a teenager can be emotionally challenging. Consider joining a support group or speaking to a counsellor or therapist to help you deal with any stress, anxiety, or other emotional issues you may be experiencing.

- Educate yourself about your birth options: Talk to your

doctor about different birth options, such as natural birth, epidural, or caesarean. Understanding your options will help you make informed decisions about your labour and delivery.

- Educate Yourself: Learning as much as you can about pregnancy, childbirth, and parenting can help you feel more confident and prepared. Read books, attend classes, or talk to other moms to gain knowledge and insight.

- Prepare for breastfeeding: Breastfeeding can be challenging, but it's also a great way to bond with your baby and provide essential nutrients. Consider taking a breastfeeding class or speaking to a lactation consultant for more information.

- Child Care Plan: As a teenage mom, you may have to balance school, work, and parenting responsibilities.

Make a plan for childcare, whether it's with family, friends, or a daycare centre.

Being a teenage mom doesn't define you, and you can still have a bright future. Remember that every pregnancy and birth is unique and it's important to work closely with your doctor to ensure a safe and healthy experience.

Chapter 4
Financial Planning for Teen Moms

As a teen mom, financial planning is critical to taking care of herself and her child. In this chapter, we explore the steps you can take to prepare a budget, find sources of financial aid, and plan for your financial future.

Make a budget

Making a budget is the first step in financial   pay stubs or other documents that prove your income. To keep track of your spending, you can use a budgeting app or spreadsheet to record your bills and other expenses. It's also important to account for irregular expenses, such as car repairs or medical bills, when setting aside money in a savings account.

When determining your spending priorities, it's important to prioritise your basic needs, such as housing, food, and transportation. You may need to work in other areas, e.g. For example, entertainment or dining out, and cut back to keep your budget running. It's also important to keep savings goals in mind, such as setting aside money for emergencies or education. To create a budget you need to:

- Track your income – This includes any money you earn from a job or other sources, such as child support or government benefit

- Track your spending – This
  includes all your bills like rent,
  utilities, groceries, and
  transportation.

- Determine your spending
  priorities: Determine which
  expenses are essential and
  which can be reduced or
  eliminated.

- Make a plan – Use your
  income and expenses to
  create a budget that allows you
  to meet your basic needs while
  saving for the future.

Find sources of financial aid

There are many sources of financial help for teen moms, but it's important to research the eligibility requirements and application process for each program. Some programs, like TANF and SNAP, have income and asset limits, while others require you to meet certain education or training requirements. Programs like Temporary Assistance for Needy Families (TANF) and the Supplemental Nutrition Assistance Program

(SNAP) can provide financial assistance and food assistance to eligible families.

- Nonprofit Organisations: Nonprofit organisations can also provide financial aid, but it's important to research the organisation and make sure it's in good standing before applying for help. Many nonprofit organisations also offer additional services, such as counselling or vocational training, to support teen mothers. Many nonprofit organisations provide financial assistance to low-income families, such as B. Help with rent or utility bills.

- Scholarships and Grants: There are many scholarships and grants specifically for teen moms seeking education or training.

- Employment Programs: Programs like Job Corps or

YouthBuild provide job training and employment support for young adults.

Plan your financial future

In addition to creating a budget and finding funding sources, it's important to plan for your financial future.

Planning your financial future will help you achieve long-term financial goals, such as buying a home or saving for retirement. It's important to start planning early and seek resources and support to help you reach your goals.

Saving for emergencies is an important first step in financial planning. Experts recommend putting three to six months of living expenses in a savings account to cover unexpected expenses like car repairs or medical bills.

Educational planning is also important for achieving long-term financial goals. Whether you plan to attend college or earn a professional degree, it's important to research the cost of education and look for scholarships and grants that can help cover costs. You may also consider starting a 529 college savings plan to save for your child's education.

Obtaining and building credit is also important for accessing loans and credit in the future.

Finding A Balance: School, Work And Parenting

Being a teenage mama is a gruelling and demanding part that takes a lot of time and energy. As a teenage mama , balancing academy, work, and parenting is important to ensure you can take care of yourself, your child, and your future. Here are some tips that can help you find that balance.

1. Prioritise your responsibilities: As a teenage mama , you have numerous responsibilities, including

minding for your child, going to school, and perhaps work. It's important to prioritise your responsibilities and concentrate on the most important tasks first. This could mean putting schoolwork ahead of social exercise or spending time with your child rather than hanging out with buddies.

2. Develop a routine: Creating a routine can help you manage your time better and balance your responsibilities more

fluently. Create a schedule for your day-to-day activities, including academy, work, and time with your child. Stick to your routine as much as possible, but be flexible if unanticipated events arise.

3. Use your support system: You do not have to do everything on your own. Your family and buddies are there for you. They can help you with childcare, transportation, and other tasks that can make it easier for you to balance your duties.

4. Look for resources: There are numerous resources available to

teenage mothers, including parenthood classes, counselling, and financial aid programs. Use these resources to complete your tasks and overcome challenges.

5. Take care of yourself: As a teenage mama , it's important to put your own good first. Make time for self- adequacy activities similar to sports, pursuits and spending time with confidants. By taking care of yourself, you can better manage your responsibilities and be a better parent to your child.

Remember that balancing academy, work and parenting is a process and it may take time to find what works best for you. Be patient and stay positive.

Chapter 5

Dealing with society's judgement and stigma as a teen mother

Being a teen mother can be judged and stigmatised by society. It can be difficult to deal with, but it's important to remember that you are not alone and there are ways to deal with this stigma. Here are some tips for dealing with social judgement and stigma as a teen mom.

1. Find a support system: Finding a support system made up of friends, family, or teen moms who understand your situation can help you deal with prejudice and stigma. They can provide support, encouragement and advice on how to handle difficult situations.

2. Educate Yourself: Educating yourself about teen pregnancy and parenting can

help you feel more confident and prepared to deal with social judgement and stigma. Examining the statistics and facts about teen pregnancy can help dispel negative stereotypes and misconceptions.

3. Focus on achievements - Focus on the positives and achievements you have achieved as a teen mother. Celebrate your achievements, big or small,

and remember that you have the power to achieve your goals by being a good parent.

4. Practice Self-Care: Self-care is important for maintaining mental and emotional well-being. Make time for activities that bring you joy and relaxation, and prioritise your physical health as well.

5. Stand up for yourself: Don't be afraid to stand up for

yourself in the face of criticism and stigma. Deal with negative stereotypes and misconceptions, speak up, and speak up for yourself and other teen mothers.

6. Get professional help if needed: Counselling or therapy can help you deal with prejudice and stigma in society. A psychotherapist can provide help and guidance in dealing with difficult emotions and situations.

7. Remember Your Worth: Remember that your worth as an individual and as a parent is not determined by your age or circumstances. You have the ability to be a good parent and achieve your goals, and you deserve to be treated with respect and dignity.

Dealing with social judgement and stigma as a teen parent can be difficult, but it's important to remember that you're not alone and there are ways to deal with that stigma. Finding a support system, educating yourself, focusing on your achievements, taking care of yourself, advocating for yourself, seeking professional help when you need it, and remembering your worth will help you build resilience and confidence despite judgement and stigma.

Building A Healthy Co-parenting Relationship With Your Partner

As a teen mom, building a healthy co-parenting relationship with your partner can be challenging, but it's vital to your child's well-being. Here are some tips to help you navigate co-parenting and build a healthy relationship with your partner:

1. Establish open and honest communication: It is important to be open and honest in

communicating with your partner about your feelings and expectations. Be sure to discuss how you plan to raise your child and what roles each of you will play.

2. Respect each other's boundaries: It's important to respect each other's boundaries and parenting styles. If you have different parenting styles, try to find a compromise that works for both of you.

3. Consider your child's best interests: Always consider your child's best interests and prioritise their needs. This means putting aside your differences and working together to create a stable and loving environment for your child.

4. Be flexible: Being a parent is a full-time job and it's important to be flexible with your partner when it comes to parenting responsibilities. If your partner needs help with anything, be

ready to step in and offer support.

5. Seek Outside Help: If you're struggling to build a healthy co-parenting relationship, consider seeking outside help from a counsellor or mediator. They can provide you with the tools and resources you need to build a successful co-parenting relationship.

Remember, building a healthy co-parenting relationship takes time and effort, but it's worth it for your child's well-being.

Chapter 6

Caring for a baby as a teen mama

As a teen mum, minding for an infant can be gruelling . But with the right support and knowledge, you can give your baby the nutrition she needs to thrive. Here are some tips for minding your baby. invigorated care feeding, sleep and rest babies generally should be fed every 2 to 3 hours and should be fed as demanded. Breastfeeding is recommended as it provides your baby with essential nutrients and strengthens the vulnerable system. However, if breastfeeding is tough, bottle feeding is allowed. It's important to make sure your baby latches on rightly and gets enough milk to avoid dehumidification and malnutrition.However, see a lactation adviser or doctor If you need help breastfeeding.

Sleep and Rest
Babies generally need 14 to 17 hours of acceptable sleep each night. They don't sleep well at first

and frequently wake up to eat and change. It's recommended that you put your baby to sleep to reduce the threat of unforeseen child death patterns(SIDS). shroud the lights and minimize noise to produce a peaceful resting terrain.

Honeycomb

Babies have small bladders and bowels, so they need frequent diaper changes. It's important to change diapers as soon as they're bemired to help with diaper rash and infections. To save Money, consider using washable diapers Instead of disposable diapers. We recommend using soft baby wipes and diaper rash cream to help Irritation.

How to deal with bellyache and other problems

Bellyache

Bellyache is a condition in which a baby cries for a long period of time, generally further than three hours a day and at least four days a week. Try swaddling a colicky baby, using a anodyne, using white noise, or carrying them in a carrier.However, see a Doctor, If your baby continues to cry exorbitantly. The cause of bellyache is unknown, but it generally goes down on its own in many months.

Other challenges
babies can develop other problems similar as constipation, burping, and rashes. It's important to see your paediatrician if your baby shows signs of discomfort or illness.

Vaccination, Illness Prevention and Child Protection

Vaccinations are a crucial part of protecting children against a variety of serious and sometimes life-threatening diseases. Vaccines work by stimulating the body's immune system to produce antibodies that can fight the virus or bacteria that causes the disease. Vaccinations should be given on a recommended schedule, usually starting in infancy and continuing into childhood.

In addition to vaccination, the prevention of diseases is an important aspect of keeping children healthy. This includes encouraging regular hand washing, practising good hygiene and teaching children to cover their mouths when they cough or sneeze. It is also important to keep sick children away from school or daycare to avoid spreading the disease to others.

Child protection is another important aspect for the safety and health of children. This includes identifying potential household hazards, such as sharp edges, choking hazards and toxins, and taking steps to mitigate the risks. Child protection can include installing safety gates, securing cabinets and drawers, covering electrical outlets, and anchoring furniture to walls to prevent tipping accidents.

When it comes to parental controls, it's important to be proactive and thorough. This means regularly checking the house for potential hazards and making changes if necessary. It is also important to keep a close eye on children, especially in the early years when they are most vulnerable to accidents and injuries. By taking steps to get vaccinated, prevent illness, and childproof the home, parents can help keep their children healthy and safe.

Developmental Milestones

Track your baby's growth and development

Supervision

It's important to monitor your baby's growth and development to make sure he or she's reaching milestones. This includes tracking weight, height, and head circumference, and tracking motor, language, and social development. Regular visits to your paediatrician can help you keep track of these milestones.

Milestone

Babies develop at their own pace, but after a certain age you can anticipate some milestones. For example, babies at 3 months can raise their heads and chest while lying on their tummies, and at 6 months they can sit on their backs. By 12 months, utmost babies can stand up and say many words with support. It's important to remember that every baby's development is different and do not compare yourself to other babies. As a teen mama , it's important to have the support of family, buddies, and community resources to ensure the best possible care for your baby. Consider joining a support group for teen mothers or seeking help from a social worker.

Chapter 7

Maintaining Mental Health as a Teen Mom

Being a teen mom can be a demanding and overwhelming experience. It's important to prioritise her psychological health so that you can give the best care for your baby. hitherto, here are some tips to maintain your internal health.

How to deal with stress and anxiety as a mom

Stress and anxiety are common among new mothers, especially teen mothers floundering through puberty. As a new mom, it's normal to feel stressed-out and anxious at times. Especially when it comes to overpowering the challenges of parenting and dealing with the stressors of teenage life. Still, it's important to find ways to manage these passions so they do not grow overpowering. Some fresh ways to deal with stress and anxiety include Practising awareness ways like deep breathing, contemplation, or yoga. Practise tone- care, like taking a warm bath or reading a book. Take a break and ask your family and musketeers for help.

Dealing with postpartum depression as a teen mama

Postpartum depression is a form of clinical depression that affects women after labor. It's estimated that 10 to 20 new moms witness postpartum depression, with symptoms ranging from mild to severe. PPD can occur at any time during the first cycle after giving birth. PPD signs may include heartstrings of sadness, irritability, guilt, hopelessness, fatigue, loss of interest in exercise, trouble sleeping, and changes in appetite. Women with postpartum depression may also find it delicate to bond with their children, and they may feel overwhelmed or worried about their capability to watch for their babies. Trouble factors for postpartum depression include a particular or family history of depression or other mood dis-temperatures, stressful life events, problems with gravidity or labour, lack of social support, and hormonal changes.

It's critical to seek medical attention if you substantiate symptoms of postpartum depression. This is especially important for teen mothers, who are at increased trouble for this condition due to the added stress and obligation of motherhood. Remedy options for postpartum depression include talking capsules, drug, or a combination of both. Cognitive behavioural remedy has been shown to be effective in treating postpartum depression, while antidepressants may be specified in some cases. Still, it's essential to weigh the implicit benefits and risks of medicine, especially if a woman is breastfeeding. Other self- care measures that can help ease the symptoms of postpartum depression include getting regular exercise, eating a healthy diet, avoiding alcohol and drugs, and getting cornucopia rest.However, calling a extremity hotline or other emergency services is vital, If you find yourself in a emergency and need immediate backing. Seeking professional help for internal health issues is a sign of strength, not weakness. Teenage mothers floundering with stress or depression should not stagger to seek help from their croaker. Healthcare providers can put them in touch with therapists or counsellors, while public health conventions or home health centres can offer free or low- cost services. Online support groups for teen mammies or mums with postpartum depression can also be a helpful resource. Remember that taking care of your internal health is just as important as taking care of your baby's physical health. Seeking help and support when demanded can help you become the smart parent you can be to your child.

Chapter 8

self- care for teen mothers

Self- care is an important aspect of maintaining physical and emotional health for teen mothers. It's important to make self- care a precedence, indeed when time and resources are limited. Here are some tips for practising self- care

- Make Time for Yourself: It's important to sculpt out time for yourself each day, indeed if it's just a lot of twinkles. This can include taking a comforting bath, going for a walk, or meditating. Try to find exercise that brings you joy and help you feel refreshed.

- Practice Good Sleep Hygiene: Getting enough sleep is important for physical and emotional health. Try to establish a bedtime routine that helps you wind down and relax before sleep. This may include avoiding screens before bed, reading a book, or taking a warm bath.

- Exercise Regularly: Exercise is a great way to reduce stress and ameliorate overall health. Indeed if you do not have access to a gym or equipment, there are numerous ways to incorporate physical exercise into your day, similar to taking a walk or doing yoga.
- Eat Nutritious Foods: A healthy diet is important for physical and emotional

health. Try to incorporate a variety of fruits, vegetables, whole grains, and spare proteins into your menus. It's also important to stay doused by drinking water in abundance.

- Seek Support: It's important to have a support system in place to help you navigate the challenges of parenthood as a teenager. This can include family members, musketeers, or support groups.

- Practise awareness: Awareness is a practice that involves being present and completely engaged in the current moment. This can help reduce stress and ameliorate overall well-being. awareness ways may include contemplation, deep breathing, or body reviews. Set Realistic aims Setting realistic aims can help you stay motivated and concentrated on achieving your dreams. Try to break larger pretensions into lower, more manageable ways, and celebrate your accomplishments along the way.

- Exercise Gratitude: Rehearsing gratefulness can help shift your focus from negative studies to positive ones. Try to take time each day to reflect on the things you're thankful for, no matter how small they may feel.

In conclusion, practising self- care is pivotal for teen mothers to maintain physical and emotional health. By making time for themselves, rehearsing good sleep hygiene, exercising regularly, eating nutritional foods, seeking support, rehearsing awareness, setting realistic pretensions, and rehearsing gratefulness, teen mothers can ameliorate their overall well- being and be better equipped to handle the challenges of parenthood as a teenager. It's important to seek out coffers and support to help navigate the complications of self- care and prioritise their own necessities alongside the demands of their children.

Chapter 9

Building a Support System as a Teen Mum

Being a teen mum can be a challenging experience, but building a strong support system can help you navigate the ups and downs of parenting.

Tips for building a support system

Connecting with Other Teen Moms

Connecting with other teen mothers can be a great way to find support and understanding from others who are going through similar experiences. You can find other teen moms through online communities or social media groups, or by attending parenting classes or support groups in your community. Sharing your experiences and learning from others can help you feel less alone and more empowered as a parent.

Many communities offer resources and support for teen mothers, including parenting classes, counselling services, and financial assistance. Research what resources are available in your community and take advantage of them. You can also look for support groups specifically for teen mothers, where you can connect with other moms and find advice and support.

Building a Strong Relationship with Your Family and Friends

Your family and friends can be an important source of support as you navigate the challenges of parenting. It's important to build strong relationships with those who are closest to you and who can provide emotional support, practical help, and guidance when you need it. Be open and honest with them about your experiences as a teen mom, and let them know how they can help.

Here are some ways to strengthen your relationships with family and friends:

- Communicate openly and honestly with them about your needs and challenges.
- Ask for help when you need it, whether it's with childcare or emotional support.
- Spend quality time with them, whether it's going for a walk or having a meal together
- Show appreciation for their support and let them know how

much you value their help and encouragement.

Building a support system as a teen mum can help you feel more confident and capable as a parent. By connecting with others, finding resources in your community, and building strong relationships with family and friends, you can create a network of support that will help you thrive as a parent.

Chapter 10

Parenting Styles For Teen Mothers.

Parenting as a teen mom can be challenging, as it often balances the responsibilities of parenting with the demands of growing up and navigating adolescence. Here are some parenting styles that can help teen moms:

1.Authoritative parenting: This parenting style is characterized by setting clear and consistent boundaries, as well as being responsive to the child's needs. It contains a balance between firmness and warmth and promotes open communication between parent and child. This style is often associated with positive outcomes in children with Increased self-confidence and better academic performance.

2.Permissive Parenting: This parenting style is characterised by being tolerant and forgiving towards the child's behavior. Permissive parents often treat their children warmly and lovingly but may find it difficult to set clear boundaries and enforce rules. This style can have the following negative consequences for children: Poor school performance and behavioural problems.

3.   Authoritarian parenting: This parenting style is characterised by strict rules and high expectations, but little attention is paid to the child's needs. Authoritarian parents are often cold and aloof with their children and may resort to punishment and criticism to control their children's behavior. This style can have negative consequences for children with Low

self-esteem and high levels of depression.

4. Indifferent Parenting: This parenting style is characterised by a lack of interest and involvement in the child's life. Uninvolved parents may neglect their children's needs and put their own needs before their children's. This style can have the following negative consequences for children: Poor school performance and behavioural problems.

In general, the most effective parenting style for a teen mother depends on several factors, including the child's individual needs and the resources and support available to the parent. It's important for teen moms to find resources and support systems, such as parenting classes and counselling services, to help them navigate the challenges of parenthood.

Chapter 11

Planning for the Future as a Teen Mum

Being a teen mum can be challenging, but it doesn't mean that you can't plan for a bright future for yourself and your child.

some tips for planning for the future:

Setting Goals for Yourself and Your Child

Setting goals can help you stay focused and motivated as you navigate the challenges of parenting. Set realistic, achievable, and specific goals. They can be related to education, career, personal growth, or any other area of your life. It's also important to set goals for your child's future, such as saving for their education or providing them with opportunities for extracurricular activities.

Continuing Your Education

High School, College, and Vocational Training, Continuing your education is an important step towards building a successful future for yourself and your child. Whether you're still in high school or looking to pursue higher education or vocational training, there are many options available to teen mothers. Talk to your guidance counsellor, research online, or reach out to community organisations to explore your options. Many schools and organisations offer flexible schedules or childcare options to accommodate the needs of teen mothers.

Building a Career and Financial Stability

Building a career and achieving financial stability are important goals for any young adult, and even more so for teen mothers. It's important to explore your options and find a career that suits your skills and interests. You can also explore ways to earn income from home, such as starting a small business or freelancing. It's also important to learn about budgeting, saving, and investing to ensure financial stability for yourself and your child.

Navigating Relationships and Dating as a Teen Mom

Navigating relationships and dating as a teen mum can be challenging, but it's important to prioritise our being and that of your child. It's important to communicate your needs and boundaries with your partner and to make sure that any potential partners are supportive of your role as a parent. It's also important to make time for yourself and engage in activities that make you happy and fulfilled.

Planning for the future as a teen mum requires effort, commitment, and perseverance, but it's essential for your success and that of your child. By setting goals, continuing your education, building a career, and navigating relationships with care, you can build a bright future for yourself and your child.

The power of resilience and perseverance as a teen mom

The journey of a teenage mother is never easy. It is full of challenges that can sometimes seem overwhelming. But as a teen mom, it's important to remember that you have the power of resilience and perseverance. By using these traits, you can overcome obstacles in your path and build a better future for yourself and your children.

Resilience is the cap potential to get better from tough situations. As a teen mom, you may face a variety of challenges, from the emotional turmoil of an unplanned pregnancy to the practical challenges of juggling motherhood with school, work, and other commitments. But even in the face of adversity, you can draw on your inner strength and resilience to keep you going. Developing a positive mindset, setting realistic goals, and finding sources of support will help you weather the storm and come out stronger on the other side.

Perseverance is the quality of persevering in the face of obstacles. It is the will to keep going, even when it seems difficult or impossible. As a teen mom, there may be times when you want to give up. This is when the demands of motherhood, school, work, and other commitments seem too much to handle. But if you use your natural tenacity, you can get through the tough times and achieve your goals. By focusing on your vision for the future and taking small steps toward your goal every day, you can build the life you want for yourself and your children.

Ultimately, the power of resilience and perseverance lies within you. As a teen mom, you can take advantage of these traits and use them to overcome the challenges you face. By staying true to yourself, staying focused on your goals, and reaching out for help when you need it, you can create a bright and prosperous future for yourself and your children.

Conclusion

Congratulations on completing this guide on teen motherhood! As a teen mom, you've already overcome many challenges and have taken on the incredible responsibility of caring for your child. It's important to take time to reflect on your journey so far and to recognize all that you've accomplished.

Remember that you are not alone in this. There are many other teen mothers out there, and there are also many resources available to help you navigate the challenges of motherhood. Don't be afraid to reach out for support when you need it, whether that's from family, friends, support groups, or professionals.

As you continue on your journey, here are a few pieces of advice to keep in mind:

1. Take care of yourself: As a mother, it's easy to put your child's needs ahead of your own. However, it's important to prioritise your own physical

and mental health so that you can be the best possible parent for your child.

2. Celebrate your successes: Being a teen mom is hard work, and you should be proud of all that you've accomplished. No matter how small your success may seem, celebrate them

3. Keep learning and growing: As your child grows and develops, you'll also have new challenges to face. Keep learning and growing as a parent so

that you can continue to provide the best possible care for your child.

Finally, know that there is hope for your future. While being a teen mom may present unique challenges, it's also an opportunity to grow and learn in ways that you may never have imagined. With hard work, determination, and support, you can create a bright future for yourself and your child.

Reflecting On Your Journey As A Teen Mom

Becoming a teen mom can be a difficult and overwhelming experience, but it can also be a time of growth and learning. It takes courage and resilience to face the challenges of parenthood at such a young age, and I encourage you to embrace that responsibility.

As a teen mom, you've probably had to balance the demands of parenthood with the challenges of completing your education, pursuing a career, and managing your social life. This can be a lot to handle, and it's understandable if you've encountered obstacles along the way.

It's important to acknowledge the progress you've made on your journey as a teen mom. You may have developed strong time management skills, learned to prioritise your tasks, and gained a greater appreciation for the value of family and support.

Of course, there may have been difficult moments, such as Feeling isolated or overwhelmed, facing criticism or judgement from others, or struggling with financial or emotional stress. It's important to recognize these challenges and seek support when you need it, whether it's from friends or family, joining a support group, or seeking professional advice.

As you move forward, know that being a teen mom doesn't determine your future or limit your potential. With hard work, determination, and a support network, you can achieve your goals and build a bright future for yourself and your child.

Don't forget to celebrate your successes, learn from your mistakes and keep growing and learning on this journey.

Advice For Teen Mums

If you are a teenage mom, here is some advice that may help you on this challenging but rewarding journey:

- Find support: Parenting can be overwhelming and it is important to have a strong support system. Reach out to friends, family members, or organisations that support teenage parents.

- Prioritise your education: Education is not only important for your future, but also for your child's. Find out about opportunities to complete high school or pursue higher education, such as B. Online classes, flexible schedules, or child care assistance programs.

- Take care of yourself: It can be easy to neglect your own needs when you are focused on caring for your child. Don't forget to take time for yourself to rest, relax and pursue your interests. This will help you maintain your well-being and be a better parent in the long run.

- Build a strong relationship with your child: Bonding with your child is critical to their development and well-being. Take the time to play with your child, read to them, and be present in their lives.

- Don't Let Others' Opinions Define You: There may be people who will judge or crib size you for being a teenage mom, but remember that their opinions do not define you. Focus on your own goals and values and surround yourself with people who support and encourage you.

- Set goals and work towards them: It is important to have purpose and direction in life. Set goals for yourself, whether it's completing your education, advancing your career, or building a stable home for your family. Take small steps toward those goals every day and celebrate your progress along the way.

Remember that being a teenage mom isn't easy, but it's not a barrier to success either. With hard work, determination, and support, you can build a bright future for yourself and your child.

Encouragement For Teen Moms

As a teen mom, it's important to know that you have the potential to achieve great things in the future. Despite the challenges you've faced, you've already shown incredible strength, resilience, and dedication in raising your child.

With hard work, determination, and a support network, you can achieve your goals and build a bright future for yourself and your child.

Don't forget to celebrate your achievements, no matter how small they seem. Even if you encounter setbacks or obstacles along the way, know that you have the strength to overcome them.

It's also important to seek out support and resources to help you achieve your goals. Many organisations and programs assist teen parents, such as B. Childcare, learning resources, and counselling services.

Most importantly, remember that you are not alone. Many other teenage parents have had similar experiences and can offer advice, encouragement, and support. Keep going, stay focused on your goals, and believe in yourself. With hard work and perseverance,

you can create a bright future for
yourself and your child.